Back on the Basketball Court with a Smile

A Case for Vision Therapy

By
K. Joseph Hill

Copyright © 2018

ISBN: 978-0-9860254-3-3

Library of Congress Control Number: 2017919488

Published by Pacific H&L Publishing

Author: K. Joseph Hill
Cover Illustration by: Pens and Beetles Studio (pensandbeetles.com)

First Edition Published date: January 2018

Printed by Bookmasters
30 Amberwood Parkway
Ashland, Ohio 44805

All rights reserved. No part of this book may be reproduced or transmitted in any form or by any means, electronic or mechanical, including photocopying, recording, or by any information storage and retrieval system without written permission from the author except for the inclusion of brief quotations in review.

Printed in the United States of America

Table of Contents

Warm-Up v
    Thank-Yous v

Opening Quote vii

Preface ix

First Quarter: Setting 1
    Testing Day 1
    Imagine the Following 2
    Purpose 4
    In the Beginning 6
    Vision Therapy 7
    The Treatment 13
    Seeing Improvements 16

Second Quarter: Background 19
    Dinnertime Discussions 19
    Recalling the Past 20
    Returning to Play 25
    Uncle Jesse 27
    Big Sister 30

School Site: Kindergarten to Third Grade 33
Fourth Grade to Sixth Grade 36

Third Quarter: Games 40
    Game Time.. 40
    Game 1: First Game Jitters 41
    Game 2: Just Shoot the Ball 43
    Game 3: Playing Better 44
    Game 4: Level of Confidence and Aggressiveness Increase ... 44
    Game 5: Improvement with Defensive Prowess and
        Accommodative Facility 46
    Season Midpoint 47
    Game 6: Excelling at Man-to-Man Coverage 48
    Game 7: Two Unique Experiences 49
    Game 8: The Halftime Performance 51
    Game 9: The Critical Question 52
    Game 10: The Final Game 54

Fourth Quarter: Wrap Up 55
    End-of-Season Acknowledgments........................ 55
    Epilogue... 57
    Conclusion... 58

Overtime: Final Tab 63

Addendum 65

References 67

About the Author 69

Warm-Up

THANK-YOUS

Thank you to my wife, daughter, and son for understanding and bearing with the trials and tribulations surrounding our son's vision problems and supporting the process to help him see in what we deem as "normal."

Thank you to the following doctors: Dr. D. Fujimoto, OD, retired; Dr. S. Mallari, OD; and Dr. A. Lisa Fernando, OD, for their direction, support, and assistance through this experience.

Thank you to the following coaches: Uncle Jesse, Coach Gregg, Coach Marc, and Coach Matt, and parents and teammates of our Optimist Club for support and encouragement of my son in coming back and playing league basketball.

Thank you to my son's BSA Cub Pack and Boy Scout Troop.

Thank you to Mrs. Dominguez for helping me with my first book and this book.

Opening quote

"Eighty percent, approximately, of what we do in life comes through sight. If you help the most important sense, life becomes so much easier and rewarding in all other aspects of life. Your son is a success because you contributed greatly to his success. He now ranks at the top of our office's vision therapy successes, along with a young lady who once struggled with reading, but thanks to vision therapy, she is now an epidemiologist with a Ph.D. teaching at University of California Davis. She is making a tremendous difference in the lives of many."

Dr. D. Fujimoto, OD

Preface

> *"When you go, you can't take it with you. But you do take something with you: Your knowledge and skills, and wouldn't it be beneficial to share that with someone before you do go?"*
>
> John Wilson, Woodworker/Master Craftsman on a Public Broadcast Station show, 2015

I CANNOT SAY FOR CERTAIN WHAT COMPELLED ME TO WRITE THIS STORY; however, as I saw the first game unfold upon my son returning to league play in the sixth grade, it occurred to me that there could be something to this vision therapy, and if there is, shouldn't it be told?

As each game unfolded during the sixth-grade season, past memories came back to me regarding our family's—and especially my son's—experiences before, during, and after applied vision therapy. I do have to admit that Dr. Fujimoto, Dr. Mallari, and Dr. Fernando, optometrists, encouraged me to share this story because of those who suffer with (unbeknownst to them) vision problems, and to share that in those situations, like my son's, there are forms of treatment, and how better to communicate than through a story of a child's struggles relating to vision problems.

I share this story about my son's vision problems because I, and probably others, was not aware of vision therapy. At the time I was made aware of vision therapy, it was not well known, some doubted its significance, and some with certain vision problems were believed to be misdiagnosed as suffering from some other ailment. From my experience with vision therapy, I find that it is overlooked as a learning disability (at least in my opinion). I learned that through its application, it can reduce vision problems. I certainly hope you read my son's story from beginning to end to better understand what he went through and how he came away with a noticeable level of improvement.

I ALSO ADMIT that I wrote this story from memory and thought it helpful to use the sixth-grade basketball season as a basis to determine, if possible, a means to measure success with the application of vision therapy. Please note, several years have lapsed since my son's sixth-grade basketball season and getting this book published. My hope is that someone's child, son or daughter, can benefit from my story. And lastly, although my attempt is to communicate this story with as much detail as I can recall from memory, just know that I may have left out a few of the hurts, pains, and successes along the way, and that I may have also likely missed a thing or two in trying to convey this story about my son's struggles, hardships, and experiences.

First Quarter: Setting

"You will find as you look back upon your life that the moments when you have really lived are the moments when you have done things in the spirit of love."

Henry Drummond

TESTING DAY

Upon concluding the extensive eye exam, the optometrist and my wife had the following conversation:

"Ma'am, has your son ever played baseball?"

My wife replied, "Yes, why?"

The optometrist then asked, "Has he ever hit a baseball?"

To which my wife responded, "Well, basically, no, why?"

The optometrist then went on to say, "That doesn't surprise me, and I can tell you why. Your son is suffering from convergence insufficiency, accommodative infacility, and pursuits. In other words, simply put, your son's eyes are not working properly." As a parting comment to my wife, the optometrist said, *"It's likely without vision correction, he will never be able to drive a car."*

So begins vision therapy. Before delving into this story and what vision therapy is, imagine the following scenarios, which are some of what my son experienced before the application of vision therapy.

IMAGINE THE FOLLOWING . . .

Going to the playground as a little kid and not being able to run, jump, or play on the playground equipment because, unbeknownst to you, your vision problems affect your judgment on how to climb, slide, or jump around on each apparatus.—Dismay, ouch!

Having a parent use math flash cards in order to help improve your proficiency and speed in addition, subtraction, multiplication, and division, and because, unbeknownst to you, you cannot readily focus your eyes quickly as the cards are held up, you struggle to read the cards but you can't.—Anxiety, ugh!

Being in the first, second, and even third grade, and given homework assignments that should normally take anywhere from 30 minutes to 2 hours at most, but because, unbeknownst to you, you have vision problems, your homework takes up to *5 hours* to complete! Your parents become frustrated with you, yet they try to do their best to extend their level of patience, help, and understanding.

Being a child able to watch other children your age learn to ride a bicycle or a scooter, but because, unbeknownst to you, you have vision problems, you cannot rid yourself of bicycle training wheels nor find the means to balance yourself on the scooter.—Frustration meltdown!

You're on the basketball court and your teammate calls out your name to pass you the ball, then throws the ball to you, but because, unbeknownst to you, you have vision problems, you cannot react in time to catch the ball, and it winds up smacking you in the face.—Ouch!

You're on the basketball court and a teammate bounce passes the ball to you and because, unbeknownst to you, you have vision problems, you misjudge the ball, and it goes right by you. Your teammate calls out to you in a stern voice, "Hey, you should've caught that!"—Emotional distress!

Imagine, unbeknownst to you, you have vision problems. It is difficult to perform these typical early childhood activities, so you slide into levels of emotional unhappiness, frustration, depression, anxiety, and social withdrawal. However, confusing the issue is . . . *you can see!*

Imagine complaining about having migraine headaches, so you visit your general medical doctor, who finds nothing out of the ordinary that is causing problems (even knowing that vision problems can cause headaches). You have had your routine eye exam and you are wearing corrective lenses, but still, occasionally, more frequently it seems, you suffer with headaches. Certainly not a good feeling.

Cumulatively, the straightforward signs of vision problems for our son were: headaches more frequently, long hours of doing homework in early elementary school grades, not being active in physical activities, plus showing signs of frustration when attempting to do physical activities, not doing well with simple computer games, not being able to ride a bike or scooter, and difficulty in dealing with and judging visual distances and moving objects.

Yes, there were other situations that could be added, but the above does give a good overview of situations experienced by my son. Thus comes the question, how could he experience such major difficulties even though he was fitted with glasses? He could make out people, objects, and things around him, including the ability to see planes flying high in the sky, and yet, he still struggled with the situations noted above. A good question. I hope I can shed light on it through the following story.

PURPOSE

The purpose of this book is to tell the story of one child's experiences in dealing with undetected vision problems in his early adolescence to overcoming such deficiencies. The vision problems that afflicted my son early on affected his abilities to perform or do well in school, sports, and other typical activities that young children involve themselves in. Simple activities such as: riding a bike or scooter, playing computer games, or interactive children's games were not easy for him. The telling of this story is to hopefully help others to possibly identify and subsequently deal with vision problems not of the norm such as typical nearsightedness and farsightedness. I share this story, in part, from a sports perspective due to the fact that as my son's sixth-grade basketball season progressed, past issues and problems, coupled with present success with vision therapy, became very apparent to my wife and me.

I begin this story by indicating that I have written this book from my chronicling my son's sixth-grade-level basketball season, which, as the season unfolded, a flood of memories and experiences came well to the forefront of my mind so that I felt compelled to write this story. It is my hope through sharing my son's story and reflecting upon prior to, during, and postseason basketball play, that it will enlighten others in recognizing and dealing with children who may suffer with vision deficiencies that are of the same or similar nature to my son's vision deficiencies.

My wife and I had no idea of the extent of his vision problems until we fully understood what his identified disorders were and how severe they were in terms of how it affected him. For our son, and likely others, what makes this a difficult situation is that he had no barometer to measure or contrast his vision by how good it is (or not), and thereby at a young age, be able to communicate something is not right because, with emphasis, he only sees the world through his own eyes, and as we know, one cannot contrast and compare it with others' except through proper testing.

It is believed that one out of five children have some form of vision deficiency, and such vision deficiencies could be mistaken for some type of learning disability. It should be noted that although vision problems such as my son's are not deemed to be a learning disability—but in my opinion, they should be—they can mimic such learning disorders as ADD, ADHD, dyslexia, Asperger's syndrome, and other forms of learning disabilities (*New York Times*). I begin this story with this: I am not a doctor of any type, nor do I profess to be an expert in the field of human vision, eye care, vision therapy, or anything related to these topics. What I *can* say and share is that by observing my son's struggles with school, sports, and general physical activities, and discovering vision therapy, I believe I can communicate an experience that, in turn, may help others.

To further this, I am taking the liberty of shedding some light on this subject so that when it comes to basic education, learning, playing sports, or other physical and interactive activities, that a child that has trouble with or struggles in these areas that may very well be deemed to be associated with vision problems, that it doesn't label him or her as one who can't play a sport, can't learn, can't interact socially, etc. Where the application of vision therapy could reduce or eliminate problems associated with such, that as time goes by, it helps them accelerate in these areas as has been noted by different sources citing such testimonials from vision therapy application (Judith Warner, *New York Times*) rather than they become labeled as lazy, unable to learn, socially dysfunctional, etc.

IN THE BEGINNING

"You hear with your ears, but you listen with your eyes."
                                        Coach Mike Bokosky

Coach Bokosky said this at a youth basketball clinic where my daughter and I attended. He went on to say that if you focus your eyes on the person speaking, or on the activity unfolding before you, or things happening around you, you will learn. If you don't use your eyes to focus on them, then you will tend to wander off—in a daydream state—and thereby miss the point of the story, or instruction being given, or the message being communicated. He said he strives to instill in his players that if you focus your listening with your eyes, you *will* learn.

What I came away with that day was his quote that stuck with me and came to resurface in my mind in looking at my son's struggles with school, homework, sports, and other activities. I felt that there may very well be something tied to his inabilities in relation to his vision. My son's struggles with these things included extremely long hours just doing homework in grades one through four, his inability to ride a bike or a scooter, or even show a level of playing ability in team sports with children his age. So began the road to discovering his vision problems.

Another aspect in pursuing trying to understand what was causing my son such difficulty with various aspects of school and homework, sports, and general activities (things that pertained to eye/hand coordination and depth perception) was something that my optometrist indicated to me years earlier. When my daughter, who is 4 years older than my son, had an eye exam when she was 7 or 8 years old, our optometrist, knowing my daughter had an interest in playing sports, suggested that if she pursued sports and I felt she had an issue with eye/hand coordination, to bring her in and be tested for such. And if there was such a deficiency, then apply the appropriate vision therapy program(s) that would help her. Fortunately, as time went by, my daughter showed no signs of needing vision therapy. However, later, I recalled her comment about eye/hand coordination testing and wondered if it might apply to and be beneficial to my son.

VISION THERAPY

"It is the spur of ignorance, the consciousness of not understanding, and the curiosity about that which lies beyond, that are essential to our progress."

John Pierce

What is vision therapy? you may ask. Certainly, neither my wife nor I had any knowledge of it. Vision therapy is basically a program that works the various eye muscles in a way so that they can function normally. The program, depending on the degree of vision problems, can include computer applications, printed chart exercises, and other physical exercises to enable the eyes to work properly.

For my son, his vision deficiencies were identified as convergence insufficiency, accommodative infacility, and saccades and pursuits. Rather than labor here with an in-depth medical definition of these terms, below, I share a generalized brief overview of each one that I garnered from the Internet as I understand them to relate to my son's conditions, but I would say in general terms that my son's eyes could not track a moving object coming toward him or away from him. He could not readily focus on close objects, and then on faraway objects clearly and quickly. He also had significantly reduced depth perception. These are what my son was identified with, but note that there are other eye deficiencies such as "walled eye" where the eye drifts out or away from the other eye, sometimes called "lazy eye." Different Web sites delve in-depth on vision therapy and vision-related problems and issues. I would also point out a book, noted below, that I found very helpful in understanding this field of vision therapy.

Convergence insufficiency. This relates to eyestrain, double vision (diplopia), blurred vision, and/or headaches. This is a two-eyed vision disorder that does not allow the eyes to work with close-up work easily. It is this disorder that affects coordination, sports, judgment of distances, and possibly even motion sickness. Convergence insufficiency may go undetected in school-age children even if they pass a simple 20/20 eye exam. Specialized testing for convergence insufficiency has to be performed in order to determine its existence (Optometrist Network).

Accommodative facility. This affects the vision that does not allow the eyes to focus clearly when quickly looking at close objects, and then faraway objects. Most people can see clearly in focusing on objects both near and far and vice versa in about one-fifth of a second. This situation relates to sitting in a classroom and looking at your notepad/paper on your desk, and then looking up to take notes off the chalkboard. Looking far, and then near intermittently is easy for most people, but for those affected by this dysfunction, their eyes struggle to focus on one or the other, or possibly both. Even with corrective lenses, the problem is not resolved. Other complaints related to this include discomfort in tasks that demand visual interpretation such as use of flash cards, making errors in copying notes onto paper from the chalkboard, and even reading material close to the face or having one's face very close to the desk surface (guthrieeyecare.com).

Saccades and smooth pursuits. Saccades is a small rapid jerky movement of the eye especially as it jumps from fixation on one point to another (as in reading), where the eyes move across sentences and experience jerky reading, causing one to lose one's place while reading, and/or missing a word(s) (Dr. Sue Fowler). Pursuits refers to your eyes tracking moving objects that move in space, like watching a ball being thrown from one person to another as in playing catch. (Our optometrist indicated our son was experiencing pursuits as one of his problems.) These two can be combined as symptomatic, and it

First Quarter: Setting

is further noted that some who suffer with saccades and pursuits can also experience convergence and divergence, and accommodation problems/issues. Again, some of these symptoms can reflect poor eye/hand coordination, inability to track objects, and a lack of coordination and clumsiness (visiontherapycenter).

I will not go in-depth regarding the many facets of vision therapy. A well written book titled *Eye Power, An Updated Report on Vision Therapy*, by Dr. Stan Appelbaum and Ann Hoopes, 2009, illustrates, discusses, and covers the various aspects of vision awareness and related matters concerning this topic of vision therapy. The book is well written and goes into detail about vision therapy, the types of vision problems identified for treatment, related topic statistics, studies conducted on the subject matter, and case examples of effective treatment. It is important to note that according to the authors of this book that there are believed to be too many young children that are misdiagnosed with ADHD, when their real problems were deemed to be vision related, even if the individual was found to have 20/20 vision. They also point out that many years ago, little credence was given to this application of vision therapy. Only recently is there a greater understanding of these problems and application of this subject (Appelbaum and Hoopes 2009).

At around 4½ years old, my son has had to wear bifocal corrective lenses. The upper portion of the lens was prescribed for his nearsightedness and a lesser prescription for near activities was prescribed for the lower portion of the lens. The bifocals were to slow down his jumps in nearsightedness. So very early on, he has had to wear glasses for vision deficiencies that typically don't occur in most children until later in their adolescence or teen years. You may ask why then wasn't he caught with his vision therapy problems as early as 4 or 5 years old with these early eye exams. I will share Dr. Mallari's observations on this, which sheds some light on this question. Her observations on the matter are very insightful and worth noting.

According to Dr. Sharon Mallari, typical routine eye exams do look for convergence/divergence, accommodation, ocular mobility, strabismus, and the like. However, to a certain degree, the patient plays an important role in this exam. The patient needs to communicate their visual experiences so the examiner can check further if something is out of the norm. Unfortunately, young children don't fully understand whether they are having any type of vision problem(s) beyond nearsightedness and farsightedness testing. This is where parents need to share observations about their children's experiences, such as struggling with schoolwork, physical activities, and other activities that depend on vision. Dr. Mallari notes that teachers, coaches, and others should share their observations with the parents. What happens in certain exam situations, as expressed by Dr. Mallari, is that children want to show their parents that they can see, but in reality, most young children cannot relate vision problems beyond the basic understanding of seeing near and/or far. Typically, children want to do well in front of their parents in exam situations and unless parents inject such observations and issues as those noted above, symptoms go unannounced and thereby possibly do not get detected early (Dr. S. Mallari).

Although the presumption is that vision issues should be picked up during routine eye exams and the parents should not have to ask for additional testing, it may take a combination of input from the child, parents, and the optometrist, if further testing is needed. However, as Dr. Mallari notes, vision therapy screening is an additional cost above routine eye exam charges, which I can certainly attest to. I am not aware, at this writing, of insurance companies picking up the cost of vision therapy (Dr. S. Mallari).

Dr. Mallari also adds that a teacher and school performance play a huge part in vision issues that relate to learning disabilities. She notes that some children are labeled as having a learning disability, and depending on private versus public schools/school district, they

First Quarter: Setting

can get therapy sessions through them. However, most are private pay. If everything is fine during the routine exam, but the patient still has problems doing schoolwork, then further testing is likely needed and referral to a specialist occurs. Then the exact problem can be pinpointed (Dr. S. Mallari).

Even though my son did have eye exams once a year, since the age of 4½, why then was it not discovered that he had vision problems as I noted earlier? His eye exams were thorough, it was discovered that he needed corrective eyewear, and there were no signs of further concerns. Therefore, from our experiences in this matter, combined with conversations with Dr. Mallari, I would encourage the reader to make a special note of Dr. Mallari's two points noted above: "One, a young child is not likely to know of vision problems to further express concerns of things going on in their world," and two, "It takes us parents, teachers, coaches, and others to share observations of problems and issues with vision-related matters when it comes to children." Dr. Mallari's second point is where I have to admit that neither my wife nor I communicated such vision deficiency issues and problems in the early eye exams to the examining optometrist. Had we put together the correlation between our son's issues and struggles with vision-related problems early on and communicated them to our optometrist early on, I know for certain that she would have immediately directed us to have the proper testing done, as she ultimately did at age 8½ years old. So to answer the question why my son's deficiencies were not picked up earlier, in part, it was because we didn't communicate our observations. Parents play an important role in a child's eye exam.

Asking the question of why our son was not identified with visual problems from another angle as to why possibly we didn't communicate that information is that this is where I would say the age-old adages such as: "putting two and two together," "seeing the forest through the trees," "connecting the dots," and "had I known then what I know now," etc., scenarios come into play. I would say in part to answer this question from another angle puts a confusing spin on it with looking at the scenarios I note at the beginning of this book under "Imagine the Following . . ." For example, knowing that my son got his yearly eye exams, he could identify planes flying high in the sky, he didn't have a problem with walking to school, climbing stairs, riding a toddler's bike with training wheels, identifying people, objects, and he basically appeared to do other things visually related, so how could one know to connect the dots, so to speak, with the types of vision problems he was experiencing? Visually, to us, the parents, nothing seemed out of the norm as far as we could tell. Therefore, we could not communicate vision-related problems when not knowing they could—and—did, exist. Even though the visual problem signs were there in front of us, we just did not recognize them as such and therefore, could not communicate our observations to the examining optometrist early on. And it may be that these vision-related problems don't crop up and become apparent and/or amass more frequently until children are a little older, and things start occurring, which bring forth such issues. I believe had my wife and I become aware of vision-related problems as identified in Dr. Appelbaum's book, as found on the Internet, and so forth, it is likely we would have communicated the observed problems earlier than when we did.

Then comes the follow-up question as to at what point did I come to realize it was time to have the conversation about our son's vision deficiencies with our optometrist. This I will answer later in the story, but it resulted from a certain incident.

I do want the reader to know, however, that our family optometrist, who I have been a patient of for over 32 years (we as a family are still patients of this optometry office), was always very thorough in her exams. Our optometrist not only did standard routine checks for typical vision deficiencies for corrective eyewear if necessary, but certainly went further with the exams to check and look for other eye concerns such as glaucoma, cataracts, increases in eye pressure, looking inside the eyes for other potential problems associated with the eye (eye dilations), and usually spent an hour with her patients to not only get to know them, but become aware of family history with vision-related matters and to look for such in her patients. She also would disseminate up-to-date eye care information relating to diet, nutrition, medications, etc., and other pertinent vision-related matters such as using UV protection eyewear while out in the sun. Her approach to the practice of optometry generally was putting her patients first, staying up-to-date with the latest applications for eye care and vision treatment, as well as maintaining the office with the latest technological advances in related equipment.

THE TREATMENT

> *"Once you agree upon the price you and your family must pay for success, it enables you to ignore the minor hurts, the opponents' pressure, and the temporary failures."*
>
> Coach Vince Lombardi

The application of vision therapy prescribed for my son was a series of computer exercises working the eye muscles in order to make the eyes work in the deemed "normal" way eyes are supposed to work. The actual computer application consisted of a program that had several eye exercises, that was to be performed 6 days a week for an average duration of almost an hour each time. This initial application of 6 days a week lasted over the next 9 months. When I went on the Internet to look up additional information about vision therapy, I found several testimonials that confirmed that the normal time length for the applied therapy sessions lasted from 9 to 12 months to complete the basic vision therapy.

In doing the first 6 months of the computer-based eye exercises, we would have to watch over him to ensure he was doing each program and doing it properly. It was a learning curve for my wife and me as we assisted and watched over him. My son needed our assistance in doing a couple of the eye exercises where special glasses were used. These glasses were referred to as "flippers." We would have to flip them in a semicontinual motion while my son worked the keyboard as it applied to the particular exercise. The "flippers" act like weights during the exercises and force the eyes to struggle and work harder in order to ultimately get stronger working eye muscles.

It was difficult for me to describe exactly what the actual computer-based eye exercises were that were assigned to my son. However, as best as I can explain, they were like computer games that primarily either had objects/symbols moving around the screen, rotating objects/symbols using quadrants, and objects moving apart or together, and each one would require that you use the mouse or the directional arrows on the keyboard.

At first, my son thought it was like a game typical of computer games and didn't mind doing it. But over time, typical of things that are redundant activities for kids, it became tedious for him, at best, and irritating and annoying, at worst. He got to the point where he was not so fond of doing this 6 days a week. My wife and I had to encourage him to keep at it and explain to him the long-term benefits of vision therapy. Yes, this is a rather difficult task to explain all this to a young child. And all the while, either my wife or I had to be there overseeing that he was doing all the exercise programs as assigned to him for his particular vision problems.

In addition to the computer program, there was also a wall chart exercise that my son had to perform. This was more of a static exercise where he would have to look at a letter chart placed on the wall about 10 feet away from him and hold a letter chart in his hands, and as quickly as he could, read a line of letters on the wall, and then

First Quarter: Setting

quickly switch to the handheld one and read a line of letters from it. The purpose of this was to work the eyes in order to see far and near with quick focus adjustment of the eyes. In part, this exercise is as if you are sitting at your desk in class and taking notes from the chalkboard (or dry erase board), and then transferring the information onto your notebook paper on your desk. It involves looking up and away at a distance, and then down at your paper, which is very close to you, a back-and-forth-type motion, seeing far, and then near quickly.

To most people, this is a simple matter; to my son, however, this would take longer because his eyes couldn't focus near and far quickly, although if he stared at one or the other long enough, it would eventually come into focus (or we were of the belief it would come into focus). However, his lengthy duration isn't the norm with typical vision. It takes him so long to focus. Most people can transition with focusing near and far in about one-fifth of a second. It would then take him longer to do in-class assignments, something we were not aware of until we applied vision therapy. Do keep in mind how would a young child struggling with this possibly know that he or she is having vision problems when the child doesn't know what is "normal"?

For the first few months of applied vision therapy, we saw no improvement in my son in what he was dealing with, but we all felt we might see light at the end of the tunnel if we had him complete the program as prescribed. This was because the computer-based program had built-in scoring that could track a patient's progress. So by the sixth month, we could see that the scoring assessments on the computer showed signs of improvement. Through this vision therapy computer program, the optometrist was also able to track his progress. By the ninth month, the examining optometrist indicated that my son could reduce the number of days per week and reduce the duration of a couple of the exercises. Eventually after 12 months, he was able to reduce the exercises down to 1 day a week for about 30 to 40 minutes, depending on how long he took doing the particular exercises. At this juncture, it was presumed that my son would have to continue with this exercise program well into adulthood in order to maintain the level of vision improvement that he achieved. We will have to wait and see.

Although my son was allowed to reduce the number of days per week and lessen the duration of a couple of the computer eye exercises, after 12 months of vision therapy, what were the results? Did we see a much-changed, new-and-improved little boy? Our response was no, not really. The optometrist assured us that there was vast improvement in his vision and that we just initially don't see it. In other words, where was that *aha!* moment for us to say, *Yes, something has occurred! There are results!* But where were they? When would we see them surface?

There was no insurance to cover the cost of the vision therapy program nor the cost of several office visits associated with doing vision therapy that we were aware of. Even so, it did not deter us from seeking remedies to our son's vision problems.

SEEING IMPROVEMENTS

> "The farther back you can look, the farther forward you are likely to see."
>
> Winston Churchill

When the improvements in my son's vision started showing, a multitude of things occurred in his life. We didn't experience that sudden *aha!* moment that some may expect to come from by laboring through vision therapy, especially after 12 months of application. It was more a slow, gradual process where we didn't have that one occurrence "jump" out at us. I am sure there were little signs along the way, but initially, nothing really stood out for us that said, "This is it, this is that moment."

First Quarter: Setting

FROM MY PERSPECTIVE, in tying the success of vision therapy to various aspects of his youth, it stemmed from my looking back at my son's past and present experiences in playing Youth League Basketball to contrast "before and after."

Improvements in his vision became obvious not long after he joined a local troop of the Boy Scouts of America. He initially joined the Cub Scouts halfway through the fourth grade, and then moved onto the Boy Scouts in the latter part of the fifth grade. At first, my wife and I were hesitant to have him join any organization at that point in his life. The reason we were hesitant was due to our observation of him in how he struggled with school, sports, and other activities as I mentioned earlier, like riding a bike, a scooter, doing educational games on the computer, and generally any other activity using eye/hand coordination. He became hesitant to participate with others in those activities at school and other places. However, it wasn't without total disinterest because he looked up to his sister and wanted to follow in her footsteps with things like playing sports, learning to swim, and to do things she did. Unfortunately, he had always struggled with these various activities, only to become disinterested in them, whereas other children seemed to be picking up interest in these various types of activities.

From the age of 5 to 8, my son played youth basketball, only to find himself not doing well at it, which disillusioned him. He came to the point that he didn't want to play anymore regardless of what anyone said or did to encourage him.

That aside, we took serious consideration of what Coach Paul Thomas said at one of our Optimist Club's Scholarship Awards Banquets. He said, "If you join an organization, join one that is of good character, good morals, and good standing in the community, and encourages goodness among its members. Such as the Optimist Clubs, Boy and Girl Scouts, Boys and Girls Clubs, and the like because these organizations typically have creeds, mottos, oaths, and provisions that promote good character building, encourage giving back to the community, and are typically supportive of those around them in a positive light."

What stuck with my wife and me from listening to Coach Thomas was that if we could have our children in such organizations, regardless of their personal deficiencies, it would help them in some way go down the right path of life. So again looking for any opportunity to help our son in what he was struggling with, we allowed him to join scouting.

Our initial concern with him joining the Cub Scouts was that he would become disillusioned with that as well. We felt his take on what he thought would be something that he would enjoy and have fun with probably would not be like that. He asked that he be allowed to join, but again, we were hesitant, fearing that it would turn into what he had been experiencing with all the other things up to that point in his life . . . that he would become frustrated, disinterested, and further withdraw from the other children and activities.

We gradually became involved in the local scouting program, and my son seemed to take a liking to it. He developed friendships and actively participated in the different Cub Scout activities without showing signs of frustration and disappointment in himself on how well he could perform/participate in those activities, regardless of the activity. I believe improvements in his vision allowed him to better see what other kids were doing in the same way other kids were seeing the "world," so to speak. In turn, this evidently was not the case prior to vision therapy, and now it may be seen as him being on the same level as most other children vision-wise.

From the Cub Scouts, he moved into Boy Scouts, and this is where the results of vision therapy came to light. Not only were the signs coming to light within my son with school, sports, and activities, in general, but for us, his parents, as well.

Second Quarter: Background

"Grown men can learn from very little children for the hearts of little children are pure. Therefore, the Great Spirit may show to them many things in which older people miss."

Black Elk

DINNERTIME DISCUSSIONS

Joining the Boy Scouts led my son to come back and play basketball, where, again, earlier, he would not have been interested.

What typically occurs in our house at dinner is what teachers and educators urge parents to do at the dinner table, and that is to ask your children what they did that day, and specifically, what they did at school. About the time my son was in the fifth grade, he would come home with scraped elbows and knees, and at the dinner table, we would ask him about his day at school. He usually wasn't much of a talker, sort of quiet most times, but he would share some details of his day, although he wouldn't make mention of his scraped elbows and knees. At first, I just let it go, but as time went by, this became somewhat of the norm with him periodically coming home with scrapes and bruises. My wife and I finally had to press the matter with him and ask what was going on to cause these minor injuries. Naturally, I initially feared this problem was related to his vision problems, let alone imagining all kinds of playground scenarios typical of kids at play during recess. As it turned out, he said he was playing basketball and would occasionally somehow wind up scraping the blacktop during these games. I asked if he was getting knocked down, slipping, hurt, scrapping elbows and the like, then why was he playing? His quick response was, "I like playing!"

So from there, I thought, would he be interested in getting back into organized play in a league suited to his caliber of play? I suggested to him that there are a couple of Boy Scout merit badges he could earn by playing in a basketball league. At first, he was hesitant of my suggestion, but with my encouragement and the encouragement of a couple of other individuals who later were to become his basketball coaches, he decided to give it a try. I believe in tying basketball back to scouting, like pursuing a certain merit badge, so I'm sure he saw that this would be of some benefit to his scouting.

From this point forward is where I really started to see his improvement, and the relationship with where vision therapy had brought him. Not only seeing the improvements, but as the season unfolded, it allowed me to reflect and thereby recall the various instances of things that occurred in my son's life, especially between the ages of 4 and 9, that I could point to the fact, again, unbeknownst to us, that he had serious vision problems. As the story moves on from here, I will not only infuse the basketball practice sessions and later share the basketball games' experiences, but I also intertwine different occurrences that further shed light on my son's struggles and difficulties with his early vision problems.

RECALLING THE PAST

> *"The greatest accomplishment is not never falling, but in rising again after you fall."*
>
> *Coach Vince Lombardi*

When I took him to the first practice of the season in his sixth-grade year, as we walked into the gym, I quickly recognized parents and children from the past, as well as some memories coming back to me

Second Quarter: Background

of my son's earlier years with this organization's basketball program and other things that are a part of this Optimist Club's activities. Where I took him to play basketball was to the Optimist Club where we had originally joined when my daughter began playing at age 7, also noting they have a little kids program, which starts at age 5. Our son began at age 5. I felt this Optimist Club was a good organization to return to, not only in regards to learning and playing the game of basketball, but as all Optimist Clubs go, it had other good attributes, such as community involvement and charitable fund-raisers.

We had our son start early, at 5 years old, believing it would help with his motor skills. He liked following after his sister who played basketball, volleyball, softball, and baseball with this Optimist Club's organized league play of each of these sports. When it came time to participate in the Saturday morning practices and games geared for their level, my son kept trying and wanted to keep coming to these practices and games, but he still showed signs of struggling with the activities. We had no inkling of what was going on with our son other than thinking maybe he just needs more time to develop, more practice, and more encouragement. This was to no avail, however. What helped to keep him coming back was that he met two other children that he liked playing with, and they would encourage him to come to the Saturday sessions and to other Optimist Club activities. What became troubling as time progressed was that he just wasn't performing at the level the other children his age were.

As parents, we were certainly not looking for our child to rise up and become a pro-ball player of any type, but at least as one who would come to play and enjoy these sports and games as they were intended for youths to experience and, hopefully, have fun with. Our primary goals for our children, aside from getting an education, were to be able to swim, ride a bike, and be able to play a team sport.

As my son grew with this Optimist Club's program, youth sports, and other activities, he would become more and more disheartened, frustrated, and even break down and cry about his inabilities as compared to the other children. What became the norm with his early experience with basketball practices was when the ball came at him, regardless of being passed to him or coming off the basket, the ball would hit him before he could raise his arms and hands to catch it. Now, imagine this continually happening, to the point that his glasses would become damaged and had to be repaired a few times. We had to invest in sturdy sports goggles with prescription lenses. At this point is where you come to ask yourself, "Why isn't he catching the ball even with these sturdy goggles?" In addition to not catching the ball readily, when passing the ball, he would have a short, weak throw, and to shoot the ball at the basket would take what would seem an eternity. To take this a step further, during the summer months, the Optimist Club would have T-ball and baseball leagues for the youth to participate in. In a nutshell, my son participated—to no avail with any type of success. He struggled to catch or hit a baseball and wouldn't throw the baseball very far.

With these observations, we wondered whether it was even safe for him to continue to participate in these sports. I also sensed other parents and coaches felt he shouldn't be out there. Certainly as a parent/coach, especially for young children, it is hard to approach someone and say something to the effect that *your child should not be out here playing*. Most people would take offense to a comment like that about their own child. I could empathize with them. I knew I had to make a decision regardless of whether my son wanted to continue to play anymore for fear of an injury that would be labeled as a *"If you had taken him out when you suspected or felt there was something wrong, then this would not have happened"* scenario.

What I recall from the last season of basketball play before I took him out was that he would do certain things that would get him out of finishing practice, sort of self-defense mechanisms such as saying he had a headache (again, noting that vision problems can cause headaches), or somehow wind up on the floor needing my assistance

Second Quarter: Background

to pick him up and sit with him as practice continued. But one lasting recollection I had from this time was during one practice session where they were having a full-court practice scrimmage, and during this scrimmage, a teammate passed my son the ball. The ball went right past him, and his teammate said loudly, "You should have caught that!" At that moment, my son walked to the corner of the gym and broke down and cried. Then quickly, one of the coaches went to him and consoled him for several minutes. I asked the coach afterward what my son said. The coach said that my son felt his teammates didn't understand that he was trying his best. Yet, why couldn't he play as well as the other boys? Apparently his frustrations finally came to the surface as a result of this incident.

My heart went out to him. Just an 8-year-old boy so wanting to be like the others. I was perplexed and didn't know what to do. I knew he was trying his best. He wanted to be so much like the others. Even though I consoled him as best I could that day by encouraging him, like *keep doing your best, don't give up, and keep practicing; you will get there*, I knew in my mind that at this point, continuing in this program would only become more problematic for him. I believed it would possibly further lead to a decrease in his level of confidence in himself, thereby affecting future endeavors in any physical activities, let alone academic and social interactions.

The previous situation with the missed basketball pass occurred with about two weeks remaining in their basketball season. This situation just lingered in my mind. It just stayed there as some sort of signpost telling me something wasn't right. Something needed to be done as to what was going on with my son and his physical inabilities, and even the other things that were running through my head that he wasn't doing well with either. I believe it was at this juncture that I would say through an epiphany of sorts (Coach Bokosky's quote, my optometrist's comment about eye/hand coordination testing, and the like) that I came up with an idea of doing a test, if you will, with my son's ability to catch a small ball. I took a small rubber ball, one used in the game of handball, and had my son stand about ten feet away from me, and I proceeded to quickly toss the ball to him three consecutive times. Each time I tossed the ball, he missed it. I then asked after the third time, "Do you see the ball coming at you?" His reply, "No!" The next business day, I called my optometrist and shared what I did with my son using the ball, and then elaborated on other situations he was experiencing that related to vision. My optometrist immediately scheduled the extensive eye-testing exam within a few days of my phone call. And this is where "Testing Day" came about that I shared at the beginning of this story. (Please note that I do not in any way make my experiment with catching a handball as a guaranteed means of determining vision-related problems. That is best left to the professionals.)

EVEN THOUGH I took him out of the basketball program and had him stop playing with this Optimist Club's sports programs, I wasn't willing to give up on him. So, I had him keep up with his swimming lessons, which he seemed to do fine. I considered him a good swimmer. I signed him up for a couple of local recreational programs just to keep him active during the summer. Also, as part of an added level to his vision therapy, I started playing catch with him using either tennis balls or Wiffle balls so that if he didn't catch a ball with his hands and it hit him, it certainly wouldn't hurt him. I would start close and move back a few steps every so often so that it would not just help in his eye/hand coordination and eye exercises, but help build a bit of confidence in him. At first, he was not good at catching, but we kept at it, and he did start to catch the ball more frequently.

Later on, in addition to playing catch, I would also pitch to him using Wiffle balls, and he would use a light aluminum bat to hit them. At first, he would still show signs of frustration and dislike in doing this, which was evident by his demeanor, coupled with now that I understood it, his eye tracking problems. The signs were that he still was not quickly tracking the objects coming at him or gauging how far to throw the ball. And he had trouble hitting the pitched Wiffle balls. It was progress at a slow pace, and to him—not fun.

By the time he was in the fifth grade, this is where noticeable progress was being made! He became more consistent with catching and throwing the ball, as well as hitting the ball. At this point, he seemed to start liking the time we would spend playing catch and with me pitching to him. At one point he insisted on pitching to me and having me hit the Wiffle balls. At this moment when he pitched to me, throwing the balls fairly straight, accurately, with the desired distance, and for me being able to hit the ball, I believe this was a measurable moment. At this juncture is where I started to believe there was improvement with his vision. However, not having some measuring stick to measure whatever level of improvement was made to this point, I was just not quite certain to what degree improvement was made.

During this time, we would go over to the local park and shoot hoops for added activity and exercise. Doing this over the course of the fifth grade, I believe it helped him in returning to organized play. He wasn't totally devoid of any physical activity during this time, or not handling a basketball during this time.

RETURNING TO PLAY

"What you are as a person is far more important than what you are as a basketball player."

Coach John Wooden

Continuing on from the point of us entering the gym, one of the coaches that encouraged my son to come back and play several times over the past 3 years greeted him, checked to see if he had enough air in his basketball, then directed him to shoot around as a warm-up exercise until official practice began. After this greeting, I sensed that my son was hesitant about rejoining the club. I then proceeded to tell him that if he didn't feel comfortable at any point, doesn't like it, and does not want to play, I would understand, and we would leave and call it quits. I further told him that at any time during the season that if he wanted to quit, I would understand and that would be the end of it too. I said this in part because I knew this level of play for the sixth-graders started down the road of intensifying play level and skills, and knowing that my son had been away for 3 years may show in not being at the same skill level as these kids who had been continually playing in this Optimist Club. In turn, it could become a bit too intimidating for him.

I also shared with his coaches his past issues with vision problems. They understood when I told them that we were taking this one step at a time, one practice at a time, and one game at a time. In my concluding comments to them, I told them that I shared with my son that at any point, for whatever reason, he could leave and not finish out the season. Three of the main coaches for this grade level knew my son's past experiences and understood, to some degree, what he had gone through previously. The coaches said it was their season's objectives to make it fun, infuse a level of competition, increase skill level, and come away with a better understanding of the game of basketball combined with teamwork.

As my son began the season with the practice sessions, you could see that his level of play, compared to the other boys that were there, was definitely not at the same level. If they were ranked from 1 to 28 (28 was the number of boys signed up for that season), and 1 being the best, 28 being the least best, my son hovered between 27 and 28. Although that may have been an indication in comparison to the other boys, the coaches liked what they saw in him and assured me that they would work with him as much as possible to get

Second Quarter: Background

him up to speed like the other boys. In addition to typical Saturday practice sessions, this organization passed out weekly homework assignments, which was mainly practicing your learned basketball skills at home, such as dribbling, passing, shooting, and strengthening exercises. This was their way of helping the players improve their abilities between Saturday practices since they only practiced as a team on Saturdays. As a way of ensuring that he would stay focused on schoolwork, Boy Scouts, and other activities, including vision therapy, I told him he didn't have to do the basketball homework as often as prescribed.

I WOULD ATTEND most of his practices and would always ask how things were progressing—how was practice for him, any issues or concerns he experienced, and if there was anything we needed to talk about. He would generally say it was fine, no problems, he was getting the hang of it, and adjusting back into the scheme of things. Even though I did attend his practices and observed how he was doing, as well as the rest of the players, his coaches would still keep me abreast of his progress from their perspective. One coach in particular I refer to as "Uncle Jesse," would tell me how well he was doing with particular drills and plays. Uncle Jesse knew my son very well even before he started playing at age 5, and he would contrast his performance from previous years to the present. He would note how well my son had improved over the years, both physically and emotionally.

UNCLE JESSE

Uncle Jesse was one of two coaches that whenever we would cross paths during my son's 3-year absence from this Optimist Club, he would talk to my son and encourage him to come back and play, sometimes in a "colorful" way, if you get my drift. My son, on the other hand, typically wouldn't say much to Uncle Jesse because he wouldn't know what to say, and usually, my son is just a quiet person. (Uncle Jesse was not a direct relative of mine, but he seemed like an uncle to me.)

I would say Uncle Jesse was probably one of the best youth coaches around. Probably a whole book could be dedicated to him. Uncle Jesse has six children, four sons and two daughters, all of whom were very good basketball players. I'm certain he learned a lot from not just raising his children, but coaching them as well, especially in basketball. What he displayed was a means to deal with children, how to motivate them, how to instruct them, and how to get through to them. One of his approaches to dealing with the kids is to ask them what type of student they are, an "A" student or a "C" student, whether they had common sense or no common sense. He did this as an ice breaker at the start but emphasized this because this is how he would approach them in instructing them, giving them direction, and just generally, how best to coach them. It was his means of how to figure out how to deal with each player.

However, Uncle Jesse is known for being long-winded on and off the court, and during his times of long-windedness, he would infuse things in his instructions that the kids would find amusing. For example, he would yell at the kids to cut out the BS and play basketball! Then the kids would say, "What does BS stand for?" and Uncle Jesse would say, "You kids are too young for me to say what it stands for!" Then the kids would say, "We know what it stands for and it sounds so funny when you say it," so Uncle Jesse would say, "Okay," and then say, "Bull Spit!" That would make the kids laugh hysterically.

I should digress a bit here and note that while my daughter played in this organization, I helped coach her teams (basketball and baseball). I also helped coach my son's teams his first 3 years, but for his fourth season I stepped aside. During the season of basketball, Uncle Jesse would lecture us coaches about life, basketball, and other topics, even though there were female coaches present. I was probably

Second Quarter: Background

one of two coaches that seriously listened to his hour-long Saturday morning lectures before we began practice. During these lectures, I remember one coach would come in, sit down, and keep his dark mirrored sunglasses on the whole time. He would sit there very motionless, never saying a word, so we thought he napped through Uncle Jesse's lectures.

Even though I do admire and respect Uncle Jesse for sharing and infusing his knowledge and his approach to basketball and sports to the players, coaches, and parents alike, I do recall one time at the end of one of his practice sessions during this sixth-grade season, Uncle Jesse called all the players over to the side of the gym he was on, and then began one of his long lectures, which I gathered lasted about 15-plus minutes. I wasn't within earshot, so I could not hear his words of wisdom, but I was sure it was something worth hearing. When he finished, the boys gathered up their things and proceeded out of the gym. As I walked with my son to the car, I had to ask him what important things Uncle Jesse had to say. My son's quick response was, "Not much!" My reaction, "Huh?"

As the practice sessions progressed, my son gained friendships, got placed on a team, and was showing positive signs of being back on the court. Even one parent commented to me that regardless of how rough the boys got, my son would have a smile on his face! As I would watch him during practices, fearing that the past would repeat itself—breakdowns, frustration, and general disinterest in continuing to play—I saw him moving in the opposite direction. He was displaying a happier and more positive attitude, certainly not the signs of frustration when making mistakes, or not doing the drills as well as the other boys, or struggling with attempting to learn some of the basic defensive positions. He was just having a better time with it.

It should be noted that the boys that made up my son's team were generally positive and supportive of one another regardless of abilities. The boys would typically run around together before and after practices and games. I believe this interaction made it easier for my son to readjust in coming back and playing with this organization.

Before moving on with the basketball season, there are two areas that I believe are relevant and should be shared with respect to dealing with my son's vision problems and vision therapy. The first is contrasting abilities with his older sister, and the second is my son's elementary school experiences.

BIG SISTER

"Always keep an open mind and a compassionate heart."
Coach Phil Jackson

Parents often compare and contrast between their children, call it human nature, and we as typical parents did just that with our two children. Our daughter is 4 years older than our son. Therefore, he had plenty of opportunities to learn from watching his big sister do various things and activities. It was our impression that he certainly wanted to follow in his sister's footsteps. Our daughter is both academically and athletically talented. When pursuing sports, she typically performed well, quickly grasped the fundamentals of each sport, and did so even from an early age. She started in our Optimist Club with basketball and later joined in the club's other sports programs that included softball, baseball, and volleyball.

I digress again to share a story about one basketball game of my daughter's third season of playing basketball. To me, it was one of the most exciting games I had ever seen regardless of level of play. The girls started out with only six of their nine players on the roster. Three girls couldn't make it that day, and one girl came but had to leave by halftime due to illness. She was sad she couldn't stay. So we started the second half with only five players and were down by 12 points to the first-place team in their division. The girls dug deep and tied up the game with less than 2 minutes to play. Unfortunately, the other team put fresh players into the game at this point and wound up pulling away and winning by 4 points. My daughter wore her heart on her sleeve that day, cried a bit at the end, and felt bad for her teammates not winning or even leaving the game in a tie.

Why this game stays with me isn't only because it was exciting, but because of what two things my daughter did after that game. The first thing was at the following Saturday's practice where she asked us coaches and her fellow teammates to come together to share some reflections on that game. She said, "No matter win or lose, stand together as a team; we are here to enjoy and to learn from our experiences." Although she shared a couple of other observations about the game, I believe she was saying to all of us *"Don't feel bad about losing but learn from it and move on"* (something Coach Augie Garrido alludes to in his book in looking at things to learn from games, whether you win or lose).

I thought it was quite profound for a young girl to share. The second thing she did was what she said to her little brother shortly thereafter. She said to him, "I hope you have a basketball game experience like mine. I think it would be good for you." I later turned to my wife and shared what I overheard her say to our son. We both wondered if he really understood the depth of her comment. One will truly never know . . . other than realizing that there can be life-learning experiences from playing a team sport like basketball or baseball as Coach Augie alludes to.

Eventually, at age 12, she placed her emphasis on volleyball. She played club volleyball for a few years and was on her high school's varsity team, both her junior and senior years, as a starter both years. Although her high school coach said she could have played varsity her sophomore year, he felt playing junior varsity her sophomore year would better prep her for excelling on the varsity level.

Academically, she made it into the number one academic high school in the state of California. She took her share of Advanced

Placement classes and did well. She also participated in other school activities, such as the drama club and other school clubs. During her years of growing up, as can be seen by her accomplishments, she received various recognitions and accolades along the way in relation to her academic, athletic, and acting abilities.

Early on, our son always appeared to look up to her and would often want to do the things she did. He seemed to be that younger sibling that wanted to emulate the older sibling, especially in sports, as well as any general activities. As time passed, he would find himself falling short of her talents. At times, you could sense and feel a bit of sadness, anguish, and a level of depression in him. Our daughter, on the other hand, would just look at him and be perplexed. She would ask him to help her with her volleyball drills, then she, in turn, would try to help him with his basketball dribbling and passing exercises. She too would exhibit a level of frustration with him in his inability to do well. Why not, based on the old adage that boys are supposed to exhibit natural athletic abilities, including riding a scooter or bicycle? And even doing it at an early age. At one point we took our daughter aside, and to the best of our ability, explained to her that every child is different and that some children have strengths and weaknesses that are different from other children. We were trying to tell her that one shouldn't compare one child to the other.

My wife and I were no example setters when it came to this because we too fell to human nature and wound up comparing the two. We would say, "Why isn't our son like our daughter?" "Why doesn't he do things as well as she does?" However, we believe from our viewpoint, in our situation, that it probably was a wise choice to contrast and compare. It helped us push the point of trying to find out what was affecting our son in relation to these given aspects of growing up, doing what society deems "normal," such as riding a bike, playing youth sports and activities, and doing well in school.

If it hadn't been for a combination of watching our daughter excel at various things and our optometrist suggesting to have her checked for eye/hand coordination exercises due to her involvement in sports at an early age, we may not have considered vision-related problems regarding our son. Even though this played a role in helping to identify and deal with our son's vision problems leading to vision therapy, there is another aspect that should be touched on as well, and that is my son's early school years.

SCHOOL SITE: KINDERGARTEN TO THIRD GRADE

As our son began school, things seemed to appear normal. He did well in kindergarten and although throughout the school year, he may have had an occasional meltdown or two, his teacher did recognize him with a distinguished student award. At this time, he had been wearing bifocal corrective lenses for nearsightedness.

As first grade began, signs were starting to appear in relation to his vision problems. Although the problems were not quite recognizable to us, what we did notice was our son struggling with homework, math, assigned classwork using the computer, and computer learning games. Our daughter had no signs of having problems with any of these things at the early years of elementary school.

We approached the teacher with our concerns on these matters, and although the teacher did acknowledge that our son was lagging behind, especially in math, the teacher assured us not to worry. The teacher conveyed to us that it was typical for boys to lag behind in the first grade and that eventually, they would catch up. Our son passed first grade, but we were not without reservations. We even contemplated holding him back and having him repeat first grade.

Moving onto the second grade, the pattern continued. He struggled with most topic matters and took many hours to complete homework assignments, even though we did whatever we could to assist him and work with him on his schoolwork. With or without our help, homework usually took up to 5 hours to complete. I believe he labored over his homework probably because he wanted to have it done before class the next day, show he can do it, and just so he could keep up with his fellow classmates.

We again met with his second-grade schoolteacher and shared our concerns and observations. The teacher replied with "Although he's lagging behind, he is doing fine; just keep doing what you are doing." The teacher shared suggestions of various approaches to help with schoolwork, but nothing seemed to do the job. Typical of one suggestion most teachers have offered up when students appear to struggle with basic math is to use flash cards. For most children, this probably helps them, but for our son, it usually took too long to give an answer as each card was held up for him to respond. As a result, he got the answers wrong, but what elevated the frustration was that when he was asked verbally without the card held up, he usually got it correct. We also found that he was more likely to get things correct with his homework than in-class assignments and in-class tests. Now, looking back on this time, it certainly looked as though he was having some sort of vision problems.

We recognized that our son just barely kept above the overall minimum requirements to pass onto the next grade. We believed our son's first three teachers were very good teachers and were patient with us and our son. We took their advice and applied it as best we could in helping our son with his educational studies. Regardless of what advice we applied, generally, nothing seemed to improve his test scores, reduce homework time, or answer why one day he would get it right—and then a week later get the same thing wrong. His test scores mirrored a roller coaster of sorts, up and down consistently.

When our son started the third grade, we made a point at the beginning of the school year to meet with his teacher to discuss our concerns and observations with what we experienced up to that point with our son's education. The teacher was enthusiastic about beginning her first year of being a full-time teacher and liked the challenge of having a student such as ours in her class. What the teacher offered in light of our concerns, especially long hours of doing homework, was after-school homework sessions, which were an extended class day. Other students were also given this same opportunity, and according to the teacher, this certainly helped the students with getting the additional assistance they needed to better understand the subject matters being taught. This certainly made it easier on parents as well when it came to homework-related questions because the children had more time in the classroom with the teacher who is teaching the subject matter.

At first, this seemed to help, though we're not sure why, but the teacher eventually expressed to us that he didn't need the after-school assistance; he just needed time to do his homework. The teacher said he was understanding the subject matter, he was progressing well, and that it was just a situation of him having to take longer with his homework.

It was about this time, well into the third grade, when he began his vision therapy and shortly after he began it, we shared with his teacher what we were told about his vision deficiencies. The teacher appreciated the information and would take that into consideration as the remaining school year progressed. Still, homework took several hours, he still struggled, and my wife and I did what we could to help with the situation. Again, it wasn't without frustration on our part. We were a long way from seeing any results from vision therapy, and added to his homework hours, he was doing vision therapy exercises on average 50 to 60 minutes a day, 6 days a week.

We noticed that through these early years when it came to dealing with not being consistent with his schoolwork, he usually had no answer, no idea, or no possible understanding of why he struggled, or even what could be a solution. When asked of such, he would look back at us with blank looks on his face, even sometimes sad, perplexed looks on his face.

Why this perspective is important to understand is that our son saw the world through his eyes and only knew the world through his eyes. Most of us typically see the world in what we deem "normal." Our son, on the other hand, does not know what this is, not having the benefit of experiencing seeing the world in a "normal" manner. Recall that it is believed that one out of five children have some form of vision deficiency beyond the typical nearsightedness and farsightedness. So, as his vision was improving, slowly but not quite discernible to us, he was catching up to the normal grade-level proficiency, all the while still having meltdowns and blank looks on his face.

FOURTH GRADE TO SIXTH GRADE

When he began the fourth grade, vision therapy was still high on our son's priority list of things to do. Early on in the school year, the teacher sent a note home to us indicating that she felt there was something wrong with our son. We met with the teacher and at the end of an insightful conversation, she directed us to seek out a specialist to do a battery of tests to determine if he, in fact, suffered from ADHD, Asperger's syndrome, dyslexia, or some other behavioral problem such as autism. We proceeded to have a psychologist evaluate him that included an evaluation of us, the parents, us and our son together, and our son by himself. The psychologist's initial findings were basically that our son did not have behavioral problems. We shared with the psychologist our issues with our son in regards to schoolwork, sports, social interactions, and the like, and even though he understood our plight, he found nothing out of the ordinary warranting any further psychological testing or related therapy. What the psychologist was willing to offer up was creating a type of rote methodology of extracurricular assignments, just like school homework, to further work on his basic learning skills such as math, English, spelling, etc. We opted not to consider this in light of the fact that it already took him an inordinate amount of time just to do his regular homework. Why add more on top of what he already had? Do keep in mind, his vision therapy exercises.

We took the psychologist's evaluation to our son's school and met with the school site council to let them know what we had done per his fourth-grade teacher's recommendation. Meeting with the school site council was the proper protocol when a student appears to have issues or struggles with schoolwork and/or school site issues. The council, in turn, reviewed the psychologist's evaluation, and they offered up their own suggestions, which as much as possible, we applied to our son's study habits. They also conducted their own psychological evaluation of our son, and from that point forward, they said they would monitor him on how he was doing and assess his progress with things school related. Even with all this, it just didn't appear he was improving with respect to reducing homework time or even improving with respect to physical abilities or other activities (see Addendum for further discussion on this matter).

On to the fifth grade with what might be the light at the end of the tunnel regarding vision therapy. We began the year by receiving our son's STAR test scores from the fourth-grade year. The tests results primarily indicated a noticeable amount of improvement in all subject matters covered. Certainly we signed up at the very beginning of the school year with a teacher/parent meeting, as suggested by our son's fourth-grade teacher, and again, to share with the fifth-grade teacher what has transpired academically up to that point, just trying to be concerned parents. We did this, and we let them know if there was anything they needed, we were available to help.

We believed that communication between us and the teacher as the school year progressed was very important.

We actually met with two teachers that taught fifth grade. These two teachers shared their approach to teaching the students in the fifth grade from a team approach in order to best help all the students in this grade level. They not only taught subject matter but constantly compared notes on how each student was doing and determined who needed help and what would be the best approach to helping them. They believed that not all students learn the same way or at the same pace, and thus, wanted to do their part in ensuring every student was meeting, or exceeding, grade-level expectations.

As the school year progressed, we heard of very few meltdowns, an increase in academic applications, and noticed less time doing homework. Our son also showed an increased interest in sports and other activities. For example, he first took to learning how to ride a blade scooter, and then progressed on to learning how to ride a bicycle, and rode them very well. Remember, he wouldn't try this earlier when many other kids were already riding scooters and bicycles. This, to us, was seen as a big accomplishment to ride a scooter and bicycle since kids at this age were already doing it. When our son was younger, he could not ride a bike or scooter but yet he saw other kids his age riding and probably felt depressed and withdrawn around other children. One possible reason that he couldn't accomplish this activity is that he had "reduced" depth perception or the other vision deficiencies may have played a role as well. We tried to help him learn how to ride a bike but to no success. Could this example be a situation of maybe he was just a slow learner and it took him longer or he needed to wait until older to do such things? It can be argued but when looking at other aspects in his life combined with us, his parents, coming to know what his vision deficiencies were, we were of a mind-set that vision therapy was playing a big role in this accomplishment. Regardless of whether other kids made

GAME 2: JUST SHOOT THE BALL

After getting the first game's jitters out, the team came out more aggressive and played well. My son stepped up more on defense, he stole the ball once, and intercepted a pass. He was still working on his 2-1-2 zone defense positioning. Because he was one of the taller boys on the team, they had him play in the forward's position mainly on defense. What he was needing work on at this stage was keeping himself between the basket and the opponent by not letting the opponent get inside the key/painted area under the basket.

ON OFFENSE, ON the first pass to him, he again got trapped, which caused the ball to be turned over to the other team. At this point, Coach Jesse called him over and told him, "If they pass you the ball, just turn and shoot—don't try to pass, don't dribble, don't hesitate—just shoot regardless of who's in your face!" The next time he got the ball passed to him, he turned toward the basket and shot the ball! He made the shot! A big wow! From that point forward, if the ball was passed to him, he did just that, turned toward the basket, and shot the ball. Although he didn't make any more baskets in the game, he was showing good form, and I could see confidence building in him. Again, it's worth noting that a few years before it would take him awhile to shoot the ball even when aligned with the basket, which may likely have been attributed to his vision problems.

They lost 38 to 26.

GAME 3: PLAYING BETTER

"If you're not making mistakes, then you're not doing anything. I'm positive that a doer makes mistakes."

Coach John Wooden

In this game, my son started to show more confidence in himself, and although he notched up his defensive play, he was still not quite there with positioning himself on the 2-1-2 defense. His coach kept telling him to stay in the key between the basket and the opponent. He rebounded a couple of times and passed off to his teammates for them to bring the ball down the court. At this juncture in the season, the coaches were also teaching man-to-man defense. This was to be applied when the opposing team would inbound the ball. On offense, my son kept shooting the ball when passed to him, but unfortunately, no baskets. He did, on one pass to him, get trapped by the opposing team, thereby causing the ball to be turned over.

I may have been a bit skeptical at this point wondering if he liked being there or was he just going through the motions of playing basketball. I believe he might just have realized that he was seeing in himself that he was playing better than years past. However, now, he could make mistakes, recover, and move forward. I also believe this was so because he had teammates that supported one another as well.

They won 22 to 16.

GAME 4: LEVEL OF CONFIDENCE AND AGGRESSIVENESS INCREASE

As I saw each game come and go, I saw a level of confidence increase in him where he became more aggressive on the court. He would try to emulate his fellow teammates more, and he would do what his coaches asked of him. He again stepped up his game on defense, where, on man-to-man coverage, he did really well at denying his opponent an opportunity to get an inbound pass. When the opposing players tried to pass to the player my son was guarding, on several occasions, he either knocked the ball away or intercepted the pass. I shared with my son that even if he didn't steal the ball or intercept the pass, just knocking the ball away is still a desired defensive move. I also shared this as a means of encouragement because he still knew in himself that he was weak on his dribbling abilities and needed some positive reassurances. I also told him that coaches who know the game would tell you, you win on defense.

A couple of times in the game his opponent broke away on fast breaks, dribbling down the court. My son wasn't quite keeping up with the opposing player to not foul the offensive player. So Coach Jesse told him to run as fast as he could and not worry about fouling the opponent, especially on a nonshooting foul. This way, he could run with the player and probably learn how to stay with him and not foul. So from there, the next time the opposing player took off on a fast break with the basketball, my son ran right up on him and fouled the player. Although I believe he was actually trying to reach in and knock the ball away, his reaching in somehow caused the opposing player to lose his balance and hit the floor. My son went quickly over to the player and extended his hand to help him up, and he was all right. But more importantly for my son, he was trying and he was learning.

He did better on his 2-1-2 defensive positioning and got a couple of rebounds. With the defensive rebounds, each time he made good direct firm passes out to his teammates for them to move the ball downcourt, the passes were solid, the right distance, quick, and passed to the player he intended the ball to go to. Even though he was a bit younger and smaller in size compared to his current age and height, it still can be compared and contrasted with just the basics of passing a basketball to earlier times where his passes were weak, short, and took him a while to just pass the ball.

He shot the ball several times during the game, but unfortunately did not make any baskets. Even though he didn't make a single basket, he was showing good shooting form for a sixth-grader, especially not playing competitively for the past few years. I would go as far as saying he had a natural shooting form that helped in the coming years to be more effective from the perimeter (3-point high school range). Coach Jesse told him even if you don't make a basket, each time you shoot, the more you shoot, the more likely you'll make baskets.

They won 26 to 25.

GAME 5: IMPROVEMENT WITH DEFENSIVE PROWESS AND ACCOMMODATIVE FACILITY

My son's sensing for the game's defense was again coming to light. Although still learning the finer aspects of the 2-1-2 defense positioning, he did manage to pull down three rebounds. In addition, he forced two turnovers by causing a jump ball situation and had three steals. On the first steal, once he got the ball from the opposing player, in an effort to pass the ball downcourt to an open teammate, he was called for traveling. He said afterward that he was so excited about stealing the ball that he didn't realize he took a couple of extra steps.

On offense, he shot several times with no baskets. His teammates shot a lot this particular game but didn't seem to have much luck landing shots in the hoop. Unfortunately, the opposing team seemed to have more luck making their shots.

It occurred to me in watching my son steal the ball from the opposing player, with respect to a possible vision therapy milestone, a measuring point, if you will, that each time he did it, he grabbed the ball quickly from the opposing player, something very close, then passed the ball quickly downcourt to a fellow teammate, something very far. In other words, there was improvement in his accommodative facility where his eyes were focusing on something very close quickly, and then focusing on something very far quickly, which wasn't occurring with him prior to vision therapy.

They lost 32 to 25.

SEASON MIDPOINT

"It's the little details that are vital. Little things make big things happen."

Coach John Wooden

Although this comes as the midpoint of the season, I would like to comment that they would have their practices on Saturdays and games on Sundays. As each practice came and went, my son's skills were improving. Although typical of practices as any season progresses, the players usually find liking practice sessions less and less. However, this organization would make every effort possible to have the practices challenging, keep the players moving with activities, and either taught new things or reemphasized learned drills or plays. That way, practice would be over before they knew it. It also helped by having Coach Jesse there to do his motivational pep talks and express his philosophies and stories that often entertained the kids.

I note these practices because a few times they would conduct extra practice sessions that would typically be scrimmages, not doing typical drills or play setting. As I watched these scrimmages, I could see my son even becoming more aggressive in these scrimmage games and doing the little things like setting a block or a "pick" on his own in order to allow a teammate to use him as a "roadblock" so to speak, as the teammate dribbled by him. This allows his teammate to break away from the player guarding him.

I would say in addition to him developing good shooting form, in time, he also developed the ability to set good picks. It allowed his teammates to execute "pick" and "roll" maneuvers, and conversely, rarely could an opponent set a pick on him. As time moved on, he learned on his own to roll around this offense player's pick and intercept the ball handler. Another note as time progressed, when he would set the pick, he would stand there solid like a concrete pillar where the opponent would nearly bounce off him, but he wouldn't budge.

AT THESE PRACTICE sessions, Coach Jesse would tell me how much my son has changed and improved. He was glad he came back to the organization. When someone makes note of such, especially someone who never stopped encouraging my son to come back and play (i.e., give it another try), not only does it make you feel good about your decision to give it a second chance, it also means someone else wasn't willing to give up on him either.

GAME 6: EXCELLING AT MAN-TO-MAN COVERAGE

The sixth game of the season was preceded by one of those practice scrimmage sessions the night before Sunday's game. They all played very intensely in this scrimmage. My impression was that it took a lot out of their sails for Sunday's game. It seemed the entire team was off in this sixth game. For example, the center wound up with three fouls in the first 15 minutes. He had to take a seat for what seemed like a longer period of time than he normally would take on substitution in and out during the past five games. My son did well on defense, even though I felt at this stage that he still needed work on getting a good defensive position on the 2-1-2 zone defense.

AT THIS POINT in the season, the coaches were emphasizing more man-to-man defensive coverage than staying with the 2-1-2 defensive zone setup. My son seemed to excel at this and rarely would his opponent come close to getting open to receive an inbound pass. During the game, he caused two turnovers, one was on the opponent's inbounding the ball. He knocked the ball away that fortunately went to one of his teammates. The second one was when an opposing player got a rebound under my son's team basket and my son ripped the ball away from this player and shot the ball.

On offense, he shot the ball three or four times making one basket. On one of the unmade shots, he was fouled and went to the free throw line. Unfortunately, he didn't make either of the two free throw shots.

Overall, I could see improvement in his game. Continued observation of his playing now and contrasting with years past, I was becoming more of the mind-set that the application of vision therapy was having a positive effect on him.

They lost 40 to 20.

GAME 7: TWO UNIQUE EXPERIENCES

Game seven became one of those unique experiences that further help you realize how far someone has come in their efforts from the past to the present, as well as having one of those life lessons that we all experience from time to time.

My son's involvement in the Boy Scouts led him to pursue a snow sports merit badge the day before game seven. Although he earned his snow sports merit badge, he jammed his wrist averting a fall. Yes, as luck would have it, it was his right wrist, and he is right-handed. We put a wristband on so it would minimize the pain and, hopefully, allow him to play. Coach Jesse asked him why he was wearing the wristband, and my son proceeded to tell him what happened. Coach Jesse, in his unique style asked, "Is it permanent?" My son responded, "No." Then Coach Jesse said "Good, now get out there and play!" That he did.

Although he did play less this game due to his sore wrist, he was very effective on defense. The game itself was a fast-paced, back-and-forth game. The players occasionally needed breaks to catch their breath, so my son's contribution certainly helped. His defense was quite effective by denying his opponent the ball on inbounding, he stuck with his opponent on man-to-man defense, and was getting better position on the 2-1-2 zone defense. He caused two turnovers and got in the mix a few times trying to create a jump ball situation.

What was lacking in this game was his ability to shoot, pass, or dribble well with his sore wrist. During pregame warm-ups and during halftime, he tried to shoot and dribble with his left hand but wasn't having much success.

The game was very close all the way. It came down to a tie score with 30 seconds left in the game. One of our team's players was fouled in the act of shooting. He went to the free throw line to shoot two shots. The first shot went in, but the second shot balanced on the rim for what seemed like an eternity, only to fall away from the basket. The crowd let out a big *"Aaawwwwhh!"* The opposing team got the rebound, and then drove the length of the court—only to shoot and miss with our team grabbing the rebound and running out the clock.

What was unique to this game, in addition to his improved play even with a sprained wrist, was two things. First was a compliment paid to him by a parent of one of our team's players, and second was in regards to the day before's snow sport merit badge outing.

A parent who knew my son from his earlier days of playing in this organization's basketball and baseball programs came into the gym to see how he was doing. Her son was playing in the next game following my son's game. She didn't see me at first and didn't readily recognize my son. She asked a parent she knew to point out which one was my son. I was within earshot of the conversation, and the parent who pointed out my son proceeded to tell her how he has improved since his first practice of the season, how effective his defensive prowess is, and that because of his sprained wrist, his outside shooting was sorely missed. She further said he follows his shots, passes out if he gets a rebound, and is overall a needed player equally with all the other boys on the team. Certainly an elevating compliment!

The other aspect about this game was that I believe my son felt beside himself not being able to contribute 100 percent to the game due to his sore wrist. He seemed crossed with the dilemma of wanting to be with his Boy Scout troop members the day before and missing practice, and thereby furthering the matter by not being able to come to the game where he could give it his all. I sensed it was a life lesson in trying to juggle two things at one time—hoping you can—but coming away short. I should also mention that one of his coaches, Coach Matt, was a former Boy Scout and understood the situation.

They won 25 to 24.

GAME 8: THE HALFTIME PERFORMANCE

The Saturday evening before game eight, our Optimist Club participated in a halftime show at a local university men's basketball game. The club usually does this once each season where the kids, both boys and girls, from 5 years old up to the eighth grade, perform during the halftime by showing the audience the various dribbling, shooting, and passing skills, as well as fast breaks and other drills that the kids do during practice sessions. The audience typically enjoys watching the children perform.

I watched my son along with all the other members go through their routines. It was easy to see that my son still was not up to the same level as the other boys in his grade level with respect to certain ball handling and dribbling exercises. What was important, however, was that he was out there trying his best. He said coming away from this event that he really enjoyed the experience. For me, aside of just being proud of him participating and doing as well as he could, I came away with a $40 parking ticket! Who knew they would charge for parking on a Saturday evening for our Optimist Club coming and putting on a halftime show! They still wanted us to pay for parking. Go figure.

Game eight rolled in with my son continuing to show considerable improvement from the beginning of the season. He played this game knowing where to position himself on the 2-1-2 defense. Again, they used him in the forward position due to him being a bit taller than most of the other boys on the team. He continued to do well on man-to-man pickup on the opponent's inbounding the ball. At one point, however, an opposing player he was guarding got away from him, got the inbound pass, but my son was quickly on him and prevented him from dribbling. The player attempted to get around my son, but he caused the player to lose the ball.

On offense, he got off three perimeter shots but no baskets. He did get a few offensive rebounds and made good passes back out to the point guard to allow him to redirect the offense. My son stayed in the mix under the basket on both offense and defense. He did show more aggressiveness on defense and attempted to jump and block the opponents' shots. Unfortunately, he was faked on a couple of the shooting attempts where he tried jumping to block the shot, and the player put the move on him by dribbling around him.

Overall, it was a good, tight game. Unfortunately, they lost by two points.

They lost 23 to 21.

GAME 9: THE CRITICAL QUESTION

The day before game 9, the team had another intense practice session. The practice session was what I considered a *very* intense scrimmage where the players were being most aggressive, trying

Third Quarter: Games

to grab or steal the ball from the opponent, boxed out well under the basket, and ran the court on fast breaks. Everyone shot the ball as often as they could. During breaks, the players got water, and then shot free throws. The two highlights from this practice session were when one of the coaches said my son was hitting 50 percent of his free throws, which, I guess for this age group is considered good. Coach Jesse again made a comment about how my son has turned himself around from a few years ago. In addition, one parent commented to me that after all the physical intensity, my son still came off the court with a smile.

Game 9 was where my son really stepped up his game. When contrasting his first game of the season to this game, he really showed a vast improvement in his play. On offense, he was the first one to shoot the ball. Unfortunately, the ball hit the backboard, then hit one side of the rim, and then bounced to the other side, and then popped out and away from the basket. I thought for sure it was going in the hoop! He shot several times making only one basket. My son dribbled more, partly to get closer to the basket or where he wanted to shoot from the perimeter. He made several good passes. He got into the mix on both offensive and defensive rebounding. He did well on defense by staying with his opponent on man-to-man pickup and was able to intercept two passes and blocked one shot.

Although they lost this game, the team, overall, played very intensely and very well. This was another one of those games where our team's shots fell away from the basket and the opposing team's fell in to score. At one point in the game, a fellow teammate passed my son the ball, and he missed it, only to have it go out of bounds. Although it was a turnover, instead of my son reacting as he did years earlier in that one particular practice scrimmage session, he actually let it go and hustled back down the court and kept in the rhythm of the game. I know he probably didn't like missing the ball, especially causing a turnover, but it didn't appear to bother him in the manner it did years earlier.

After the game, I complimented him on his stepped-up play and after watching all this season of his game play, his improved game, I had to ask the burning question: "Has vision therapy helped you?"

His quick response was, "Yes!"

They lost 33 to 22.

GAME 10: THE FINAL GAME

The final game of the season. This game started out and ended with a lot of back-and-forth play, both teams being very aggressive. Although my son shot the ball several times, none dropped in the basket. His highlights were more on defensive prowess where he stayed with his opponent on man-to-man pickup thereby causing one turnover. He also stole the ball three times. He shifted well when the opposing team tried to set picks on him and his teammates. I note that during the season my son worked on setting picks for his teammates and did well. Unfortunately, in this game, on one of these picks he set for his teammate, the referee called it a moving screen, which, naturally, the audience abruptly disagreed with. Even I did too!

He also made three ball saves from going out of bounds; unfortunately, the opposing team grabbed two of them. Even though the team tried their best to be as aggressive as they could, they also became a bit overconfident in making tricky passes and the opposing team intercepted a few of them. Even my son tried a couple of lob passes only to have the other team grab them. Regardless of what player threw the intercepted pass, Coach Jesse would yell at them, "What color is your uniform?"

They lost 30 to 16.

Fourth Quarter: Wrap Up

END-OF-SEASON ACKNOWLEDGMENTS

At the end of the season, typical of most youth organizations, an awards banquet is held. Everyone comes to enjoy a smorgasbord of parent-made food, and the players are recognized and receive their year-end trophies and awards. Our Optimist Club has the coaches present their team to the parents/audience and say some words about each player.

In regards to my son, Coach Matt alluded to my son's defensive prowess, especially on man-to-man pickup, also that he was effective on denying the opponent the opportunity to receive an inbound pass. He also commented on how well he progressed through the season, especially being away from the game for 3 years.

As a final note on the just finished season of basketball, I wrote the following to the coaches and players' parents on my son's team after the awards banquet because I believed it to be most fitting based on what we saw with my son and how everyone was helpful and considerate of his circumstances:

"To all now that the season has ended, my wife and I would like to extend a sincere and heartfelt thank you to each of you for your support, commitment, and understanding with all involved in having a good basketball season. We certainly appreciated the efforts put forth by all and certainly the comradery that we shared. We are taking this opportunity to also say thank you to everyone for their consideration, understanding, and support in the challenge in having our son come back and play after an absence of 3 years. Although it may be to some just another kid coming out and playing, it is difficult to describe fully in words while trying to be brief in what our son experienced in the past with his first years in our Optimist Club's tinkos, peewee lowers, and peewee middle groups, and not knowing at that time, the extent of his vision problems, let alone what he has done since to improve his vision through what is called vision therapy (still ongoing at this time). Even though it took some encouragement from Jesse, Gregg, and myself to have him come back and play, we believed that in a return to play, it would be most befitting for him to play at our Optimist Club since, in part, if it hadn't been for playing in this Optimist Club youth sports program at an early age, we may not have discovered his vision problems as early as we did. Again, an expressed sincere thank you."

"These types of wins are what our Optimist Club is really about!"
Coach Gregg

"Players with fight never lose a game, they just run out of time."
Coach John Wooden

Before closing out this story, I know that even though the team ended this season with a 3-win-7-loss record, neither the other parents nor I ever felt we had a losing season. We even believe the

Fourth Quarter: Wrap Up

boys took it the same way and viewed it as a learning and growing experience that helped elevate their play. They continued to play basketball in the coming years and probably excelled as a result of their efforts and hard work they put forth during their sixth-grade season. In looking back at that season, I would like to believe that due to their comradery, each of them would have continued to play way late into the night during those Saturday night practice sessions if we parents let them.

EPILOGUE

After the end of the sixth-grade basketball season, my son continued to play two more seasons of basketball in our Optimist Club's league. During his seventh- and eighth-grade seasons, he played in several 3 on 3 and 5 on 5 tournaments. Of particular note with one tournament in which there were an estimated 1,500 participants in this 3 on 3 tournament, my son and another boy got their picture taken by a reporter from a Japanese American Los Angeles newspaper. The photo was an action photo of them. It was used to highlight an article about that particular tournament (Rafu Shimpo). Of note in this particular tournament, my son made several 3-point shots and was very aggressive with his defense. Although he improved significantly on his game as well as his overall abilities with respect to basketball, his interest in basketball waned after his eighth-grade year.

Through this time, he maintained his interest in Boy Scouts and his Junior Optimist Club activities. He also took serious interest in cycling. He found he liked cycling more than the other activities, including basketball. Uncle Jesse always said when kids reach that age of 13 or 14, they usually either stick with what they are doing or change interests and pursue something else. My son decided to pursue cycling instead of basketball.

At the end of the eighth-grade basketball season, he began preparing himself for a long bike ride with his Boy Scout troop, along with another Boy Scout troop. The long bike trip was planned to ride from Monterey, California, to Santa Barbara, California, along California Highway 1, the scenic coastal route. The ride was nearly 300 miles in length. He biked the entire distance except for 1 day of the journey due to dehydration. That day, he had to rest. Although my son did decide to step away from basketball for this long bike ride, irony would have it that one of the basketball tournaments that he really liked occurred at the same time the bike ride took place, and it was actually in one of the towns along Highway 1. He was a bit bummed he couldn't do both, although I could tell he was searching in his head if there was some way of accomplishing it.

As I STATED early on, our interest with our children, aside from education, was to learn to ride a bike, be able to swim, and play a team sport. My son has accomplished these three activities, and I would say, in part, I would have to attribute it back to vision therapy.

I leave the story here at the time my son enters the ninth grade (high school) with this antidote. As irony would have it, on the day of freshman orientation, class sign-up, etc., we were trying to find out about the school's bicycling sports program and what my son needed to take care of in order to participate. As we inquired with the vice principal/assistant athletic director about the cycling program, he shared his biking experiences and could relate to my son's type of road bike, and he further elaborated about the school's bicycling program. Ironically, his parting comment to my son was, "Did you go over to the athletic table and get yourself signed up for basketball?"

CONCLUSION

In drawing conclusions from my son's sixth-grade school year—improved academic test scores, basketball, Boy Scouts, and general

Fourth Quarter: Wrap Up

activities—I believe it can be attributed to vision therapy. I am not a psychologist, ophthalmologist, optometrist, or any other in a specialized field. I cannot with absolute certainty say that it was vision therapy that elevated my son's abilities academically, athletically, and his general activities. However, when I searched the Internet and found many testimonials to this application of vision therapy—knowing that research individuals developed programs to deal with vision problems beyond the normal nearsightedness and farsightedness, along with some writings on the subject of vision problems/vision therapy—that I would have to say there has to be a serious level of credence given to this subject matter.

I would like the reader to remember and to make special note that upon my search of this topic on the Internet, what I saw consistently was that many attributed improvements in their child's academics and athletics to vision therapy, and that, like with my son, it took approximately 9 to 12 months to experience improvements. In other words, this is not a short, quick application of overnight success, and even after this initial time period, as in the case of my son, the eye exercises continued for the next 2 years at a lesser degree of application.

I would conclude that I did see improvement in my son with respect to his growing up and dealing with all that may be typical of childhood. However, what levels of improvement I've seen in my son since early childhood through what I would have to attribute to vision therapy, I cannot, with absolute certainty, assure the reader that applying such is a cure-all for what might very well be problems, issues, shortcomings, etc., that may be of a similar reflection of my son's experiences or fall within those category range of items listed typical of persons with vision deficiencies. I will add one final particular experience that I would have to say if it wasn't for vision therapy, based on my son's vision assessment before beginning vision therapy, that he probably would not have come close to obtaining both his rifle shooting and shotgun shooting merit badges. Both of these require a level of skill, and especially for shotgun shooting, hitting moving clay disks, which certainly require good eyes to track the moving object.

I would contend, though, that as I have watched my son through these years, when I see a child continually not be able to hit a baseball, or hear other parents talk of their child in the same manner or similar manner as my son, I can't help but wonder if vision therapy is something they should seriously consider. I certainly do not want the reader to leave this story with the belief that due to vision therapy that my son is devoid of problems, has become that outstanding student (see Addendum) or exceptional/star athlete, because he has not. However, what I would hope one comes away with from this story is that my wife and I are proud of his elevated abilities—academic, athletic, and other—and we do believe he has excelled from early childhood in these areas that, in part, attribute back to vision therapy. And we, as his parents, are glad that he came back and played three seasons of basketball with our Optimist Club, joined and stayed in Boy Scouts until age 18, took on a sport of his desire through high school (cycling), and dealt with his academic deficiencies through added after-school tutorial instruction from seventh grade to twelfth grade.

As I look back at some of the things my son did and accomplished through this time to the present, like doing a 300-mile bike ride, playing better basketball, satisfying his Eagle Scout requirements, and improving his academics, to consider this same time period without the infusion of vision therapy, I have to wonder if we hadn't pursued vision therapy, where would he have wound up? To me, not a very comforting thought.

Even well after the sixth-grade season while writing this story, additional memories and scenarios still surface in my mind of situations like the ones I described at the beginning of this book. For example, when my son was about 6 years old, we went to a youth-oriented track and field meet. My son struggled to do a couple of the

Fourth Quarter: Wrap Up

events, such as the running long jump. I would have to labor here to describe, in detail, the situations, but at least know the situations resulted in meltdowns and frustration to him. Now, looking back on this track and field event, and then now knowing his vision problems, I can say again with emphasis that not having what is deemed "normal" vision really affected his participation in physical activities.

To this end, I further emphasize the point of "observations" because this is where, as Dr. Mallari says, it takes us parents, us teachers, us coaches, and others to provide, in part, shared observations and communication when things don't appear to be normal with respect to vision-related situations. Again, noting what Dr. Appelbaum indicates about persons with corrective eyewear or even with 20/20 vision, that underlying vision problems can be present and as attested elsewhere, that one out of five persons may have extended vision problems beyond the typical nearsightedness and/or farsightedness. With additional emphasis on this just from the perspectives of Dr. Fujimoto and Coach Bokosky, in their own expressed view of vision in relation to our other human senses, our vision is quite important in relation to most other things that we do on a daily basis.

THEREFORE, I LEAVE you with this:

First, my hope that parents and their children who have similar experiences like ours can benefit from my story.

Second, that the compliment paid by a parent after an intense practice preceding Game 9, "He still came off the court with a smile on his face," is likely to be attributed back to vision therapy. Doing something to put a smile on someone's face . . . doesn't that make it all the more worthwhile? And . . .

Last, as I recalled at the conclusion of Game 9 in asking my son the poignant question, "Has vision therapy helped you?" His quick reply was "Yes!" I believe that vision therapy has allowed my son to see the world as others see the world in what we deem as "normal" vision.

Overtime: Final Tab

Our daughter:
   Graduated college summa cum laude
   Maintained good standing in her college sorority
   Has six collegiate radio awards under her direction as manager of KCR college radio

Our son:
   Logged an estimated 9,000 cycling miles between the eighth grade and twelfth grade
   Earned his driver's license
   Satisfied Eagle Scout requirements
   Was accepted at four universities

Addendum

I BELIEVE IT IS IMPORTANT TO SHARE THE FOLLOWING IN LOOKING AT THE overall picture with our son in regards to academics. Although he was evaluated early on for human-related disorders/disabilities such as autism, Asperger's syndrome, or the like, and was found to be just below the line for such, he was later reevaluated in the ninth grade because there still seemed to be some struggles with his academic performance. He still, to some degree, struggled with schoolwork assignments, including not completing assignments, and had a higher degree of problems with test taking. It is important to note that this second round of assessment evaluated him using testing that was more focused on academic-related issues and found he qualified for what is called the 504 Plan. The testing determines if a child needs additional assistance with schoolwork, needs more time to complete tests or homework assignments, or other educational assistance, and if so, then help is given to the student so that the student is considered to be at a reasonable competitive level with fellow students at the same grade level.

Why I point this out is that even with vision therapy applied and completed exercises by the child, there still could be an underlying issue with a given child, as was the case with our son. Which goes back to the optometrist's contention that observation of a child by a parent(s), educators, and others in assessing what further evaluation may be needed can be critical in a child's development, and one type of application to help a child may not be the only solution.

Again noting vision therapy may not be the cure-all, but where possibly would we have gotten to if we hadn't done the vision testing early? How bad would things have gotten for our son without vision therapy? Understandably, the question with our son cannot be answered for certain due to his going through vision therapy and having success with it. But further assessing the matter does pose a plausible question or two concerning what good would it have been with either coming away with some understanding of his situation in the fourth grade, or later on, his academic-focused testing in the ninth grade if he hadn't gone through vision therapy?

One last note, it may have been too that the psychologist that evaluated our son in the fourth grade may have had the same or similar assessment with academics as was found to be the case with the second round of evaluation in the ninth grade. We just may not have understood that at the time. To note that from the ninth grade through the beginning of twelfth grade, he also received help through a private tutorial program to help and deal with his academic deficiencies, and then onto extended help with English, math, and other subjects.

References

1. Judith Warner. "Concocting a Cure for Kids with Issues," *New York Times,* March 10, 2010, http://www.nytimes.com/2010/03/14/magazine.
2. Mike Bokosky. Head Coach Men's Basketball, Chapman University, Orange California, Association of Division III, Coach of the Year 2008–2009, 2009–2010; school's overall winningest coach and serves as assistant athletic director since 2002; credited with 22 straight winning seasons, eight seasons with 20 or more wins, and has over 400 wins; won the SCIAC tournament championship game 2014.
3. Dr. Sharon Mallari, optometrist. Written communications and follow-up conversations with Dr. Mallari, May 22, 2014, September 12, and September 30, 2015.
4. Paul Thomas. Head Coach Women's Basketball at Saint Mary's College, Moraga, California. Tenth season at St. Mary's with a record of 173–116 and Coach of the Year 2014–2015; 12 seasons at California State Polytechnic University, Pomona, California, back-to-back NCAA Division II National Champions, and NCAA II Coach of the Year 2002; overall record 406–273.
5. Optometrist Network since 1996, www.optometrist.org, July 2016. http://guthrieeye care.com/care/focusing-problems/#more215, July 2016.
6. Dr. Sue Fowler, www.patoss-dyslexia.org, July 2016. http://www.thevisiontherapycenter.com/discovering-vision-therapy.
7. Dr. Stan Appelbaum and Ann Hoopes. *Eye Power, An Updated Report on Vision Therapy*, BookSurge Publishing: 2009.

8. Augie Garrido with Wes Smith. *Life Is Yours to Win*, New York: Touchstone/Simon & Schuster, 2011.
9. Rafu Shimpo. *Los Angeles Japanese Daily News,* Los Angeles, California, September 1, 2010.
10. Vince Lombardi. Quotes: 46 quotes and quotations by Vince Lombardi, http://www.brainyquote.com/quotes/authors/v/vince lombardi.html.
11. John Wooden. Quotes: 31 quotes and quotations by John Wooden, http://www.brainyquote.com/quotes/authors/j/john wooden.html.
12. Black Elk and John Pierce. Quotes: Famous quotes and authors, famous quotations for all occasions, http://www.famousquotesandauthors.com.
13. Winston Churchill. Quote: Famous quotes about vision, http://www.famousquotes.com/topic.php?tid=1277.
14. Henry Drummond. Quote: Motivation quotes, http://http://thinkexist.com/quotes/with/keyword/motivation.
15. Phil Jackson. Famous quotes and quotations at Brainy Quote, http://www.brainyquote.com.

About the Author

K. Joseph Hill is an urban planner by profession and has practiced in the field of urban planning for over 38 years. He holds two certificates in architectural technology from El Camino College, a bachelor of science degree in urban planning from California State Polytechnic University, Pomona, and a master's degree in public administration from California State University, Fullerton. He has also coached, assisted, and participated in youth sports programs and activities through a local chapter of Optimist International and Boy Scouts of America, and has authored and published a children's picture book: *Little Pineapple, the Little Hawaiian Truck Discovers the Sugar Cane Trains*, Pacific H&L Publishing.